EKG

EKG Interpretation Made Easy: A Complete Step-By-Step Guide to 12-Lead EKG/ECG Interpretation & Arrhythmias.

Eva Regan

Contents

This book is not intended as a substitute for the medical advice of physicians. The reader should regularly consult a physician in matters relating to his/her health and particularly with respect to any symptoms that may require diagnosis or medical attention.

Section 1: Introduction

The electrocardiogram (EKG) is a recording of the electrical activity of the heart over a period of time using electrodes that are placed on the body. Whatever your nursing specialty, mastering the EKG is a key skill every nurse needs to acquire in order to provide the best care for clients. EKG interpretation will enable you to take your nursing skills to the next level, from identifying life-threatening arrhythmias to being able to diagnose a developing myocardial infarction, as well as many other cardiac disorders.

For future nurses, attempting to master the EKG can seem rather daunting. To overcome this, it is crucial to come to grips with this topic and to spend enough time developing and furthering your interpretation skills. This concise preparation guide will cover all the major areas of EKG interpretation, along with the key points that you will need to know.

Firstly, you will be able to spot a normal EKG almost instantly. On top of this, the purpose of this guide is to teach you to spot and accurately interpret the abnormalities that can occur on the EKG. When interpreting the EKG, it is essential to have a systematic approach. The trick to efficiency is to follow a pattern and to get into the habit of following key steps each time you are interpreting EKGs.

The five main areas you need to master in order to be effective in interpreting EKG are: Rate, rhythm, axis, block and infarction – all of which will be covered in this guide in that order.

At the end of this guide, you will be able to confidently navigate and interpret the complex road map of electrical activity and quickly evaluate all the main pointers correctly. This will put you on a steady path to being able to recognize abnormalities early and provide the best care for your patients!

Remember that ambition is the first step to success. The second step is action – hard work and determination. Purchasing this guide is an indication of your ambition, now it's time to get to work!

Best wishes,

Eva Regan

Section 2: EKG Basics

In this section we will cover the essential theory that underpins EKG interpretation: depolarization and repolarization, and the electrical conduction system.

1. Depolarization and Repolarization

All cardiac cells are electrically polarized in their resting state, that is, they have a negative resting internal charge with respect to their outsides. This negative resting internal charge is maintained by membrane pumps that ensure sufficient negatively charged ions are kept within the cells.

Depolarization and repolarization refers to the change in the electrical charge. Depolarization is the process in which cardiac cells lose their negative internal charge. Depolarization flows from cell to cell, stripping the cells of their resting polarity, which produces a wave of depolarization that is represented on the EKG.

The cells become repolarized once the electrical conduction has come to an end. During repolarization, the cardiac cells regain their internal negativity, thereby restoring their resting polarity. This electrical activity is also recorded on the EKG.

This electrical activity which passes through the heart is represented on the EKG by the P wave, the QRS complex, and the T wave.

- The P wave represents **atrial depolarization.**
- The QRS complex represents **ventricular depolarization.**
- The ST segment and the T wave represent **ventricular repolarization.**

We will go into further detail about this in the next chapter of the book, where we will discuss the different components of the EKG waveform and what they represent on the cardiac cycle.

2. The Electrical Conduction System

The electrical conduction system is comprised of interconnected structures that allow for the passage of electrical impulses through the heart. Atomicity refers to the ability of cardiac cells to generate pacemaker impulses. Automaticity foci are the areas of cells that initiate pacemaker activity. These foci are found in the sinus node, the AV node, and the ventricles.

The Sinus Node

The sinus node is also called the sinoatrial (SA) node. Electrical activity in the heart is generated by the SA node. Below are the key points you need to remember in relation to the sinus node:

- The sinus node is the primary pacemaker of the heart.
- The sinus node is located in the high right atrium of the heart.
- The normal rate of the sinus node is 60 to 100 beats per minute.
- On EKG, sinus node activity is recorded as a **P wave.**
- A normal sinus node beat is represented by a positive P wave.

Atrioventricular (AV) Node:

Once the electrical impulse is initiated in the right atrium, it travels from the sinus node to the AV node via the intermodal pathways. Below are the key points you need to remember in relation to the AV node:

- The AV node is located in the inter-atrial septum close to the coronary sinus.
- On EKG, AV node activity is represented by the **PR interval.**

- The AV node functions as a critical delay in the electrical conduction system. The delay allows the mitral and the tricuspid valves to open and the ventricles to fill with blood before prior to systole.
- When the sinus node fails to initiate electrical impulse, the AV node can do this although only at a slower rate.
- The normal intrinsic rate of the AV node (without stimulation from the sinus node) is 40 to 60 beats per minute. This rate, in the absence of P waves, is indicative of a junctional rhythm.

Bundle of His:

The bundle of His is the distal portion of the AV node. Below are the key points you need to remember in relation to the bundle of His.

- The bundle of His connects the electrical activity from the AV node to the ventricular bundle branches.
- The bundle of His splits into two branches: the left bundle branch and the right bundle branch.
- The bundle of His is not directly represented on EKG.

Bundle Branches:

The bundle branches consist of the left bundle branch and the right bundle branch. Below are the key points you need to remember in relation to the bundle of His.

- The left bundle branch actives the left ventricle, and is divided into the left anterior fascicle and the left posterior fascicle.
- The right bundle branch actives the right ventricle.
- Both branches course down the interventricular septum and end in the apex.
- On the EKG, the electrical activity in the bundle branches is represented by the QRS complex.

In order to effectively interpret EKG, it is crucial to understand the interconnected structures that make up the heart's electrical conduction system.

3. *Review Question & Answer:*

Can you name the structures of the electrical conduction system?

1. _____
2. _____
3. _____
4. _____
5. _____
6. _____
7. _____
8. _____
9. _____
10. _____

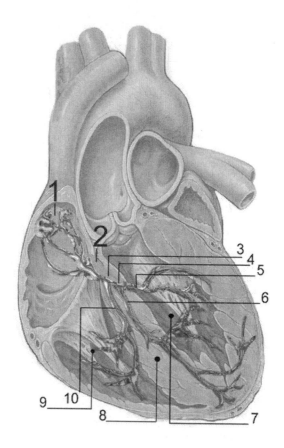

Answer:

1: Sinus Node

2: AV Node

3: Bundle of His

4: Left Bundle Branch

5: Left Posterior Fascicle

6: Left Anterior Fascicle

7: Left Ventricle

8: Ventricular Septum

9: Right Ventricle

10: Right Bundle Branch

Section 3: Understanding the Intervals

In order to accurately interpret EKG, is it crucial that you understand the different intervals and what they represent. But in order to understand the electrical conduction of the heart, it is important to briefly revisit how the cardiac cycle functions. Blood is pumped through the heart in a two-step process.

During the relaxation phase (diastole), the chambers of the heart fill with blood and then eject the blood during the contraction phase (systole). The cardiac cycle is initiated in the sinus node which causes atrial contraction. The depolarization is then delayed at the AV node but then passes through the AV bundle and into the right and left bundle branch. It is the AV node which prevents atrial and ventricular contraction to occur at the same time.

During ventricular contraction (see diagram below), depolarization moves through the heart muscle. Depolarization of the heart can be monitored and traced on EKG.

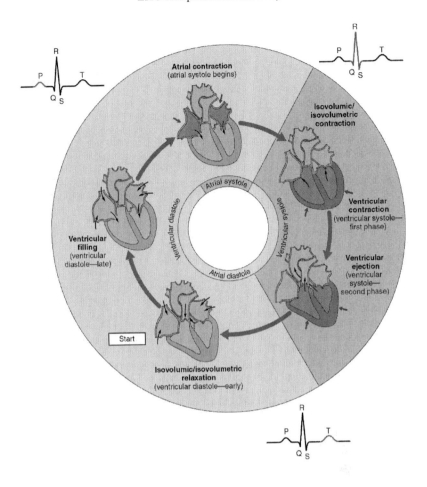

1. The EKG Waveform

Below is a brief outline of the main components of the EKG waveform. More comprehensive information on each, with their respective durations, can be found below the diagram.

The P wave: The P wave represents atrial depolarization.

The QRS complex: The QRS complex represents ventricular depolarization.

The T wave: The T wave represents the rapid phase of ventricular repolarization.

The P wave, QRS complex, and T wave are together representative of the atrial and ventricular depolarization and repolarization.

The PR segment: The PR segment represents the time between the end of atrial depolarization to the start of ventricular depolarization.

The ST segment: The ST segment represents the total ventricular repolarization time.

The QT interval: The QT interval represents ventricular depolarization and repolarization, i.e. the entire ventricular systole.

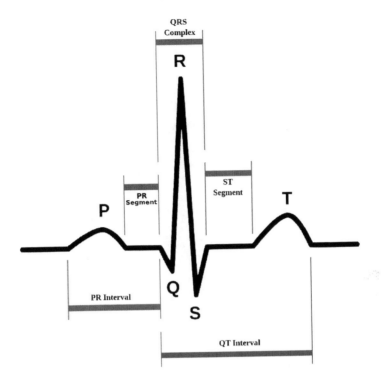

The 12-lead EKG is representative of approximately 6 seconds of time. On EKG paper, one large box represents 0.2 seconds. Each large box is made up of 5 smaller boxes which represent 0.04 seconds each.

The PR Interval: The PR interval represents the movement of electrical activity from the sinus node to the AV node. The PR interval represents the delay which is caused in order to allow blood to fill from the atria to the ventricles.

- The normal PR interval duration is 0.12 to 0.2 seconds (between 3 to 5 small boxes on EKG paper).

- If the PR interval falls below 0.12 seconds, this can be an indication of early activation of the ventrides or pre-excitation (as seen ins some forms of supraventricular tachycardia).
- If the PR interval is longer than 0.2 seconds, this is indicative of a first-degree AV block. This essentially means that the electrical conduction between the sinus node and the AV node is taking too long.
- The PR interval may also exhibit a depression below baseline which typically indicates pericarditis.

The QRS Duration: This is the duration of the QRS complex - the time that allows for the depolarization of the right and left ventricles.

- The normal QRS duration is 0.08 to 0.12 seconds (between two to three small boxes on EKG paper).
- A QRS interval that is greater than three small boxes is an indication that there is a delay in the conduction through one or both of the bundle branches.
- It is also important to note that not every QRS complex will exhibit a Q wave, a R wave, and a S wave, as can be seen in the diagram below. Capital letters represent large deflections which are greater than two small boxes. Lower case letters represent smaller deflections which are less than two small boxes. This is because the QRS interval is susceptible to all kinds of influences, including normal alterations, scar tissue, or conduction delays.

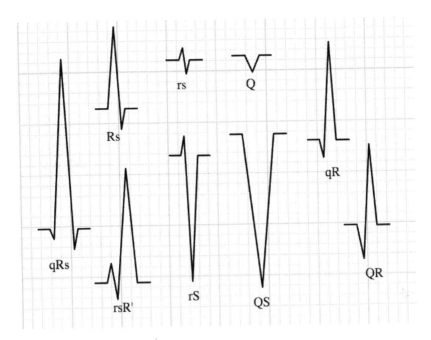

The ST Segment: The ST segment represents the beginning phase of ventricular repolarization, also referred to as the 'plateau phase'. The ST segments represents the the time from the end of ventricular depolarization to the beginning of ventricular repolarization.

- The ST segment should be flat on the baseline, or gently up-sloping.
- When assessing the ST segment, it is therefore key to look for any elevation or depression. A 2mm depression or elevation from baseline is indicative of a pathologic process.

The T Wave: The T wave represents ventricular repolarization.

- The height of the T wave is approximately one third to two thirds of that of the R wave. The T wave tends to be positive in leads with a tall R wave.
- When assessing the T wave, it is important tot note the following: a peaked appearance and inversion.
- A *peaked* T wave is an indication of electrical instability. A peaked T wave is often caused by electrolyte alterations, such as hyperkalemia.
- An *inverted* T wave can indicate an old infarction or an evolving ischemia.

The QT Interval: The QT interval represents the entire duration of the ventricular systole - the time from the start of ventricular depolarization to the end of ventricular repolarization.

- The duration of the QT interval is dependent on the heart rate. The faster the heart beats, the more urgent the need to repolarize, and therefore the shorter the QT interval. If the heart beats more slowly, the need to repolarize is less urgent and therefore the QT interval is longer.
- The QT interval composes about 40% of each R-R interval, that is the entirety of the cardiac cycle which is measured from one R wave to the next R wave.
- The normal QT interval duration is approximately 0.34 to 0.46 seconds.
- A prolongation of the QT interval is an indication of an instability in the ventricles which limits their ability to effectively repolarize. This significantly increases the risk of ventricular arrhythmias.

- Because of this, a prolonged QT interval necessitates immediate assessment. The client's medications should also be closely examined.
- Prolonged QT intervals can be caused by a variety of factors, including the following: certain drugs, certain antibiotics and antifungals medications, electrolyte abnormalities, and some antipsychotics.

The U Wave: The U wave is a deflection which can sometimes be found at the end of the T wave. An upright U wave is usually sees as a normal variant, although a great deflection can be an indication of hypokalemia or left ventricular volume overload. The diagram below shows a normal U wave in the highlighted section to the right.

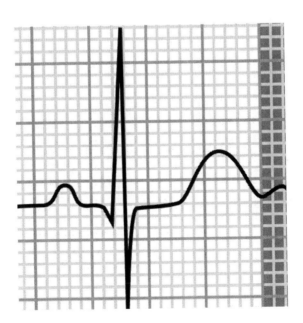

It is important to be aware of EKG characteristics relating to certain health conditions. The following is a typical example of a NCLEX-style question which every RN and NCLEX candidate should know the answer to!

2. *Review Question & Rationale*

The nurse has been assigned to a client who was admitted with gastroenteritis. Lab values reveal a potassium level of 2.9mEq/dL. Which of the following EKG findings would the nurse expect to find given the client's potassium results?

    a. A flattened QRS

    b. Absent P waves

    c. Elevated T waves

    d. Prominent U waves

Answer D is correct. EKG changes which are associated with hypokalemia include prominent U waves, peaked P waves, flat T waves, and depressed ST segments. Answers A, B, and C are all incorrect because these EKG findings are not associated with low potassium levels.

Section 4: The 12-Lead EKG

In order to record the heart's electrical activity, electrolytes are placed on the body to measure the information that we receive on EKG. The standard 12-lead EKG comprises of two lead types: chest leads and limb leads. Each of these leads has a unique angle (called the angle of orientation) from which it records the heart's activity. Because of this, it is crucial to be exact when preparing a patient for a 12-lead EKG.

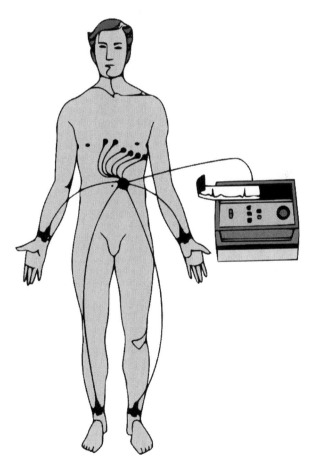

1. *The Limb Leads*

The six limb leads comprise of three **standard leads** (Leads I, II, and III), and three **augmented leads** (Leads aVR, aVL, and aVF) which are normally placed close to the wrists and the ankles. The six leads that are placed across the chest comprise of six precordial leads.

The standard leads are bipolar, meaning they have a positive and a negative pole. The standard leads record electric voltages of one location relative to another location using the left left electrode (LL), the left arm electrode (LA), and the right arm electrode (RA). The right leg electrolyte is used as an electrical grounding system.

The Bipolar Standard Leads:

Lead I: RA (-) to LA (+)

- Lead I records the electrical difference between the electrode on the left arm and the electrode on the right arm.
- Lead I is located at a 0-degree angle and is created by making the left arm positive and the right arm negative.

Lead II: RA (-) to LL (+)

- Lead II records the electrical difference between the electrode on the right leg and the electrode on the right arm.
- Lead II is located at a 60-degree angle and is created by making the leg positive and the arm negative.

Lead III: LA (-) to LL (+)

- Lead II records the electrical difference between the electrode on the left leg and the electrode on the left arm.
- Lead II is located at a 120-degree angle and is created by making the leg positive and the arm negative.

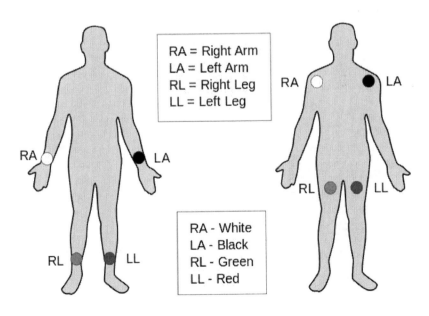

Together these three leads make up what is called the Einthoven's triangle. Summing up Einthoven's triangle, in Lead I, the left arm is positive and in Lead III, the left arm is negative, thereby cancelling one another out when added together.

To check whether leads have been correct placed, calculate whether the voltage of Lead I and Lead III equal the voltage of Lead II. If they don't, then this is most probably an indication of lead misplacement.

In order to calculate the voltage, count the number of small boxes per QRS complex. Below is an example of a correctly placed Einthoven's triangle (I + III = II):

- QRS in Lead I: 4 small boxes
- QRS in Lead II: 6 small boxes
- QRS in lead III: 2 small boxes

The Unipolar Augmented Leads:

Three three augmented leads are different to the standard leads in that one single lead is made positive and the others are made negative. Unipolar augmented leads are called 'augmented' because the EKG machine has to amplify the readings in order to be able to record them.

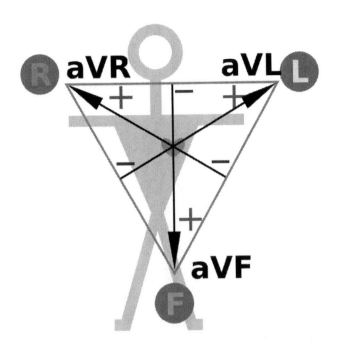

Lead aVR: RA (+) to LA (-) & LL (-)

- Lead aVR is located at a -150-degree angle and is created by making the right arm positive and the other limbs negative.

Lead aVL: LA (+) to RA (-) & LL (-)

- Lead aVL is located at a -30-degree angle and is created by left arm positive and the other limbs negative

Lead aVF: LL (+) to RA (-) & LA (-)

- Lead aVF is located at a +90-degree angle and is created by making the leg positive and arms negative.

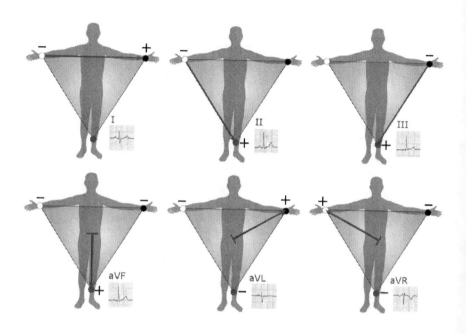

To ensure correct placement of the augmented leads, add their respective voltages together (by counting the number of small boxes). The sum should be zero (aVR + aVL +aVF = 0).

- QRS in Lead aVR: -8
- QRS in Lead aVL: +4
- QRS in lead aVF: +4

The diagram below sums up the relationship between the

(bipolar) standard leads and the (unipolar) augmented leads. This relationship defines the cardiac axis, which we will explore further in *Section 7.*

Each lead records the same electrical activity but each lead does so from a different angle of orientation. Lead II, Lead III, and Lead aVF are called **inferior leads** because they view the inferior surface of the heart (below the horizontal line). Lead I and Lead aVL are called **left lateral leads** because they view the left lateral wall of the heart.

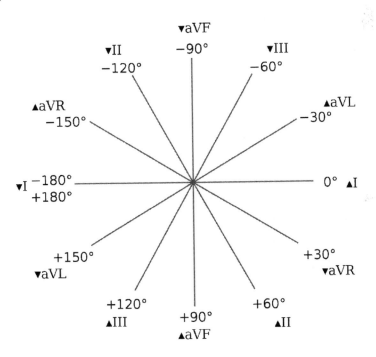

2. *The Chest Leads*

The chest leads are called precordial leads because they are placed directly above the chest close to the heart. The precordial leads comprise of six leads: V1, V2, V3, V4, V5, and V6. Like the augmented leads, precordial leads are unipolar, with one positive pole, and use a central terminal for their negative pole. The six positive electrodes are placed as follows:

- **Lead V1:** is placed in the fourth intercostal space to the right of the sternum.
- **Lead V2:** is placed in the fourth intercostal space to the left of the sternum.
- **Lead V3:** is placed to the left of the sternum, in between Lead V2 and Lead V4.
- **Lead V4:** is placed to the left of the sternum, in the fifth intercostal space sternum, on the midclavicular line.
- **Lead V5:** is placed to the left of the sternum, in between Lead V4 and Lead V5, on the anterior axillary line.
- **Lead V6:** is placed in the fifth intercostal space to the left of the sternum, on the midaxillary line.

It is important to note here that on women, leads V3, V4, V5, and V6 should be positioned just below the breast tissue, but following the same anatomical line.

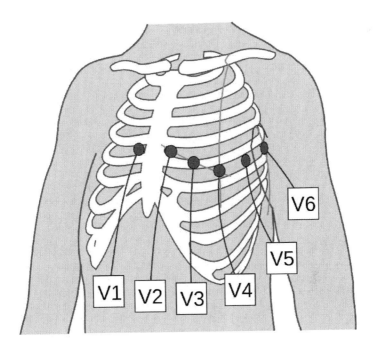

It is useful to remember the 12-Lead EKG in sets of groups because each group of leads represents a particular area of the myocardium.

Leads	Group
Leads V1, V2, V3, V4	Anterior chest leads
Leads I, aVL, V5, V6	Left lateral leads
Leads II, III, aVF	Inferior leads
Lead aVR	-

Lead aVR does not fit into any of these groups because its angle doesn't provide It a view on the left ventricle. Instead, its angle of orientation provides a view of the right ventricular outflow tract as well as the basal interventricular symptom. Lead aVR is nevertheless a very important lead to consider, especially when identifying the origin of atrial or ventricular arrhythmias.

The below diagram is a summary of the 12-lead EKG and their respective angles. It is important for the NCLEX candidate and for the licensed nurse to memorize the twelve leads, their angles, and their groups. It is also vital to remember that each lead simply records the average flow of electrical force moving within the heart at any given moment.

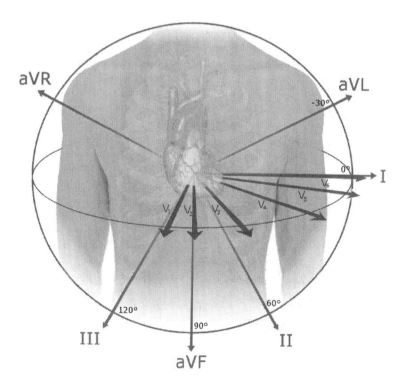

Section 5: Calculating the Heart Rate

When interpreting the EKG, it is crucial to have a systematic approach. The five main areas you need to master in order to effectively interpret EKG are: rate, rhythm, axis, block and infarction. In this section, we will cover how to calculate the heart rate.

The heart rate is easily calculated from the EKG using this simple three-step method. Firstly however, it is important to remember that one small square on EKG paper represents 0.04 seconds and one large square (made up of five small squares) represents 0.2 seconds.

Calculate the heart rate by:

1. Finding an R wave that falls on a heavy line that comprises on large box.
2. Then count the number of large squares until the next R wave.
3. Finally, count the boxes and determine the rate in beats per minute (bpm) accordingly.

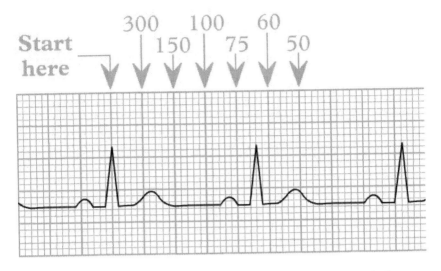

If the next R wave falls on third thick line, the client's heart bate would be 100bpm. A heart rate between 60 and 100bpm with an upright P wave indicates that the the impulse is being generated from the sinus code. If the next R wave does not fall on a thick black line, you can accurately estimate the heart rate by counting the small boxes and remembering that each small box represents 0.04 seconds.

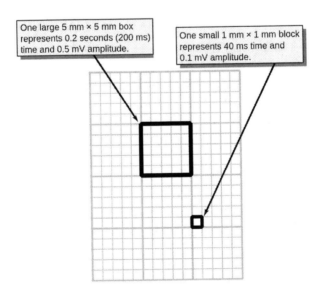

One large 5 mm × 5 mm box represents 0.2 seconds (200 ms) time and 0.5 mV amplitude.

One small 1 mm × 1 mm block represents 40 ms time and 0.1 mV amplitude.

By determining the bpm, you will also be able to identify the focus of the beat. Although every cell in the heart can technically initiate an action and stimulate the heart beat, only a few areas do so on a regular basis: the sinus node, the AV node, and the ventricles. The sinus node is the fastest focus.

- **The sinus node has an intrinsic rate of 60 – 100 bpm.**
  - o P wave present
  - o QRS interval: normal

- **The AV node has an intrinsic rate of 40 – 60 bpm**
  - o QRS interval: normal to slightly prolonged

- **The ventricles have an intrinsic rate of 20 – 40 bpm**
  - o QRS interval: prolonged

However, the slower impulse will always be overdriven by the fastest pacemaker who sets the pace. Note also that impulses which are generated from the AV node or from the ventricles will not have a P wave as the presence of the P wave indicates sinus node activity.

It is also important to note that the lower down the focus in the conduction system, and therefore the more prolonged the QRS, the less reliable and the less stable it is.

Sinoatrial node

Atria

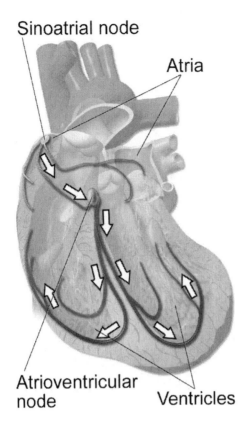

Atrioventricular
node

Ventricles

The above method for calculating the heart rate does not work for rates that fall below 40 bpm. Another way to calculate the heart rate is by following the steps below:

1. Count the 3-second intervals which you will find at the bottom of every EKG strip.
2. Count the number of cycles within to of these intervals (which will amount to 6 seconds in total).
3. Then multiply this by 10 (10 x 6 second = 1 minute) in order to accurately calculate the beats per minute.

An impulse that is generated from below the sinus node (i.e. impulses that are initiated from the AV node and the ventricles) is called a junctional rhythm. The absence of the P wave is representative of a junctional rhythm. Junctional rhythms are often related to overmedication. The nurse should therefore always examine the client's medications whenever she notes the junctional rhythm on EKG. The following medications necessitate close examination in the presence of junctional rhythms: antiarrhythmic medications, beta blockers, calcium channel blockers, and digoxin.

Before learning how to evaluate the rhythm, it is important to recap and remember the following fundamentals for the next section:

- The normal heart rate is **60 – 100 bpm.**
- A slow heart rate below 60 bpm is referred to as **bradycardia.**
- A fast heart rate above 100 bpm is referred to as **tachycardia.**

Section 6: Evaluating the Rhythm

Once you have aced your heart rate calculations, it's time to master the second part of EKG interpretation: evaluating the rhythm! In evaluating the rhythm, you essentially have to evaluate whether the QRS complex is regular or irregular. You will be able to spot a regular QRS complex almost immediately. If the QRS complexes are regular and even, then the rhythm is regular.

If there is variation however, the rhythm is irregular. A variation can be normal or pathologic. In this section, we will cover how to spot irregular rhythms and how to identify whether they are normal, abnormal and/or pathologic. The rhythm itself can be regular when it exhibits regular pattern, or regularly regular if it exhibits a repeating pattern, or irregular if no pattern is at all visible. If a rhythm is classified as irregular, it must be further classified as being either regularly irregular or irregularly irregular, which is done depending on whether there is a pattern present or not.

As a summary, a rhythm can be one of the following:

- Regular – a rhythm with a regular pattern and regular intervals
- Regularly irregular – a rhythm is regularly irregular if it exhibits some regularity to the pattern of an irregular complex

- Irregularly irregular – an irregularly irregular rhythm has no pattern at all. There are only three irregularly irregular patterns: atrial fibrillation, multifocal atrial tachycardia, and wandering atrial pacemaker, all of which will be covered in *Section 6-B.*

Sinus rhythms are impulses that originate from the sinus node. They result is a variation in the P-P interval. The normal sinus rhythm (NSR) reflects the normal state of the heart beat with the sinus node as the lead pacer.

Normal sinus rhythms share the following EKG characteristics:

- A regular rhythm with consistent intervals.
- A rate of 60 to 100 bpm
- Upright and uniform P waves
- P-QRS ratio: 1:1
- Constant PR intervals that range from 0.12 to 0.20 seconds in duration
- Normal QRS complexes that range from 0.06 to 0.10 in duration

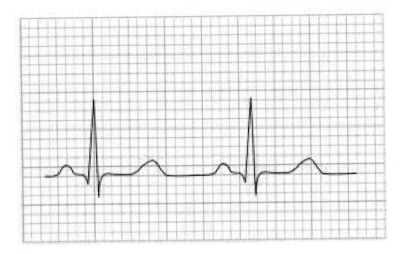

The diagram above shows the NSR. But spotting a normal EKG like the one above is the easy part. The difficulty lies in spotting and identifying abnormal rhythms. In the next three subsections, we will cover the main sinus, AV, and ventricular arrhythmias, as well as their respective EKG characteristics.

Section 6-A: Sinus Arrhythmias

The absence of a NSR is an arrhythmia, i.e. an abnormal heart rhythm. Sinus arrhythmias are among the most common irregular rhythms, most frequently seen in healthy and young people. They are a normal phenomenon caused by normal respiration that results in a variation in the heart rate which correlates with inspiration and expiration. Inspiration accelerates the heart rate (through inhibiting the vagal nerve) and expiration decreases the heart rate (which stimulates the vagal nerve). They are non-pathologic irregular rhythms and are said to be a regularly irregular rhythm.

EKG characteristics include:

- An irregular rhythm that changes with respiration resulting in differences between the shortest R-R intervals and the longest R-R intervals.
- Irregular impulses being discharged from the sinus node.
- A normal heart rate (60 – 100 bpm) which may occasionally drop below 60 bpm
- Normal P waves which are upright and uniform.
- P-QRS ratio: 1:1.
- Normal PR intervals: 0.12 – 0.20 seconds.
- Normal QRS complex: 0.06 – 0.10 seconds.

1. *Sinus Bradycardia:*

Sinus bradycardia is a sinus rhythm which is at a lower than normal rate, that is, below 60 beats per minute.

Symptoms usually arise once the heart beat falls below 50bpm and include the following:

- Chest pain
- Dizziness
- Exercise intolerance
- Light-headedness
- Shortness of breath
- Syncope

Causes include:

- Hypothermia
- Hypothyroidism
- Less common causes include diphtheria, rheumatic fever, or viral myocarditis
- Medications such as adenosine, beta-blockers, calcium channel-blocking agents, digitalis glycosides, and quinidine
- Other less common medications which can cause sinus bradycardia include
    o Alfentanil
    o Amiodarone

o Class I antiarrhythmic agents

o Clonidine

o Dimethyl sulfoxide (DMSO)

o Fentanyl

o Lithium

o Paclitaxel

o Reserpine

o Sufentanil

o Toluene

o Topical ophthalmic acetylcholine

- Sick sinus syndrome
- Sleep apnea

EKG characteristics include:

- A regular rhythm with slow impulse discharge from the sinus node resulting in a prolonged horizontal line on the baseline
- A slow heart rate that is below 60 bpm
- Normal P waves which are upright and uniform
- P-QRS ratio: 1:1
- Normal PR intervals: 0.12 – 0.20 seconds
- Normal QRS complex: 0.06 – 0.10 seconds

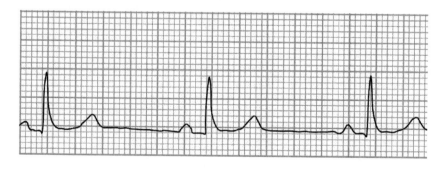

Sinus bradycardia can be normal or pathologic. Sinus bradycardia is the abnormal rhythm most commonly seen in the early stages of a myocardial infarction.

Treatment for sinus bradycardia includes:

- Administration of intravenous atropine for symptomatic clients
- Cardiac monitoring
- Intravenous access
- Provision of supplemental oxygen
- Transcutaneous pacing may be required in rare cases.

2. *Sinus Tachycardia:*

Sinus tachycardia is a sinus rhythm which is at an elevated rate. Sinus tachycardia does not usually produce any symptoms.

The most common causes include:

- Excessive thyroid hormone
- Excessive use of recreational drugs such as cocaine
- Excessive use of stimulants such as caffeine and nicotine
- Excitement
- Exercise

- Exertion
- Fever
- Hypoxia (low blood oxygen)
- Pain

EKG characteristics include:

- A regular rhythm with more frequent impulses emanating from the sinus node.
- A fast heart rate: 100 – 180 bpm.
- Normal P waves which are upright and uniform
- P-QRS ratio: 1:1.
- Normal to slightly shortened PR intervals: 0.12 – 0.20 seconds (shortens with increased heart rate).
- Normal to slightly shortened QRS complex: 0.06 – 0.10 seconds.

The EKG strip below shows sinus tachycardia with a heart rate of approximately 150 bpm.

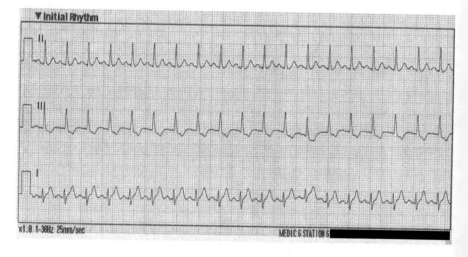

Sinus tachycardia, like sinus bradycardia, can be normal or pathologic. Treatment for sinus tachycardia is usually not required and underlying causes are treated respectively if present.

Please note that we will cover other sinus arrhythmias, including sinus pause and sinus block in *Section 8* of this guide: Heart Blocks.

3. *Review Question & Rationales*

The nurse has been assigned to a middle-aged female client. Upon assessing the client's EKG strip, the nurse notes the following findings: a regular heart rate which is greater than 100 bpm, a normal QRS complex, a normal P wave before each QRS, a PR interval of 0.12 to 0.20 seconds, and a P-QRS ratio of 1:1. Which of the following is the correct interpretation of the client's rhythm?

    a. Atrial flutter

    b. Premature atrial contraction

    c. Sinus tachycardia

    d. Sinus bradycardia

Answer C is correct. The correct interpretation of the client's EKG is diagnostic for sinus tachycardia. Answer A is incorrect because for atrial flutter, the p-QRS ratio would be 2:1, 3:1, or 4:1 and the P waves would be saw-toothed (this will be covered in *Section 6-B*). Answer B is incorrect because premature atrial complexes (PACs) would reveal variations in P waves as well as an irregular rhythm (also covered in *Section 6-B*). Answer D is likewise incorrect because the client's EKG strip reveals opposite findings – for sinus bradycardia, the clients heart rate would be below 60 bpm.

Section 6-B: Atrial Arrhythmias

Atrial arrhythmias are a common cause of irregular rhythms. They can consist of a single beat (lasting only for a few seconds) or a sustained disturbance to the rhythm of the heart beat which can last for several years.

1. _Premature Atrial Contractions (PACs):_

A PAC occurs when a cell located in the atrium prematurely triggers an impulse before the sinus node. PACs will result in irregular rhythms and often a P wave is seen before the QRS complex, although the QRS duration remains the same. PAC-caused irregularities rarely require treatment other than for symptomatic relief.

PACS are usually not a cause of concern. Treatment is usually optional as most PACs are benign. It is sometimes treated using medications such as beta blockers or calcium blockers.

- If every other heart beat is a PAC, this is called an **atrial bigeminy.**
- If every third heart beat is a PAC, this is called an **atrial trigeminy.**
- If three or more PAC's occur one after the other, this is called an **atrial tachycardia.**

Symptoms include:

- A feeling of 'missing' or 'skipping' a beat
- Palpitations
- Racing heart beat

Causes include:

- Abnormal magnesium blood levels
- Abnormal potassium blood levels
- Excessive use of stimulants such as caffeine, tobacco, or alcohol
- Hypertension
- Myocardial infarct
- Stress
- Toxicity to digitalis
- Valve disorder

EKG characteristics include:

- An irregular pattern whenever a PAC occurs which is caused by impulses being initiate prematurely.
- The heart rate is depending on the underlying rhythm and therefore varies.
- Visible P waves.
- Variations in PR intervals, i.e. in the form of different shapes: 0.12 – 0.20 seconds.
- Normal QRS complex: 0.06 – 0.10 seconds.

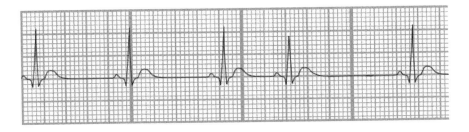

2. *Unifocal and Multifocal Atrial Tachycardia*

Atrial tachycardia occurs when electrical impulses are initiated not from the sinus node, but from within the atria at a faster-than-usual rate. It can occur in patients with normal and abnormal heart structures, as well as in people with congenital heart disease. Atrial tachycardia can be unifocal or multifocal in nature.

Unifocal Atrial tachycardia: Occurs when there is only one atrial focus that stimulates the ventricles.

- Visible P waves which are not buried in the preceding T wave
- If unifocal atrial tachycardia are non-sustained, it will cause a regularly irregular rhythm.
- If unifocal atrial tachycardia re sustained, it will cause a regular rhythm.

Multifocal Atrial Tachycardia: Occurs when there are two or more atrial foci that are stimulating the ventricles, each with a separate intrinsic rate and different automaticity.

- When there is a difference in P wave from heart beat to heart beat, this is referred to as wandering atrial pacemaker.

Both the wandering atrial pacemaker and the multifocal atrial tachycardia are common atrial rhythm disturbances. Atrial tachycardia can degenerate to atrial fibrillation (an irregularly irregular rhythm).

Symptoms of AT include:

- A rapid heart rate
- Chest pain
- Dizziness
- Dyspnea
- Fatigue
- Hypotension
- Light-headedness
- Palpitations
- Syncope

EKG characteristics of Unifocal Atrial Tachycardia:

- A regular pattern. Sinus node impulses are simply overridden by premature impulses that are fired off at a more rapid rate.
- Fast heart rate: 150 – 250 bpm.

- P waves are present and upright and uniform although they are a different shape to those generated by the sinus node.
- P-QRS ratio: 1:1.
- Shorter PR intervals of 0.12 seconds and less.
- Normal QRS complex which may be diverge at times: 0.06 – 0.10 seconds.

EKG characteristics of Multifocal Atrial Tachycardia (MAT):

- An irregularly irregular pattern
- Fast heart rate: greater than 100 bpm
- At least three morphologically distinct P waves.
- P-QRS ratio: 1:1.
- Variations in the PR intervals of 0.12 seconds.
- Normal QRS complex: 0.06 – 0.10 seconds.

The EKG below shows MAT, an atrial arrhythmia that is caused by multiple sites of competing electrical activity.

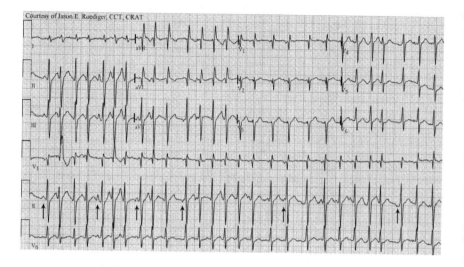

Courtesy of Jason E. Roediger, CCT, CRAT

MAT does not usually require treatment nor does it cause serious symptoms. However, if it is judged clinically necessary, the heart rate can be reduced in some cases through the administration of the following medications:

- Beta blockers and/or calcium channel blockers
- Magnesium sulphate and/or antiarrhythmic to treat multifocal atrial tachycardia

3. *Wandering Atrial Pacemaker*

Wandering atrial pacemaker (WAP), like multifocal atrial tachycardia, is caused by frequent and unpredictable beats in the atria that are discharged from different areas (foci) within the atrium. It is similar to MAT, except the heart rate is usually slower (less than 100 bpm).

EKG characteristics of Wandering Atrial Pacemaker:

- An irregular rhythm that is caused by impulses being triggered from different sites.
- Normal heart rate: 60 – 100 bpm.
- At least three different types of P waves
- P-QRS ratio: 1:1.
- Variations in the PR intervals.
- Normal QRS complex forms: 0.06 – 0.10 seconds.

Like MAT, the wandering atrial pacemaker is usually asymptomatic and doesn't usually necessitate treatment.

4. *Atrial Flutter (AFL)*

Atrial flutter is an abnormal heart rhythm which is caused when atrial depolarization occurs at a very rapid rate. In atrial flutter, the AV node is again bombarded with a significant number of atrial impulses and cannot repolarize in time for each new impulse. Because of this, some atrial impulses pass through the AV node without generating a QRS complex. Some impulses fire into refractory nodes. This is a phenomenon called AV block. The most common one is a 2:1 block, which means that one out of two flutters passes through the AV node, thereby generating a QRS complex. 3:1 and 4:1 blocks are also commonly encountered. Atrial flutter is a more organized variation of atrial fibrillation.

Symptoms include:

- Anxiety
- Fluttering chest feeling
- Palpitations
- Shortness of breath
- Weakness
- People with an underlying heart or lung disease experiencing atrial flutter may also experience fainting, chest or heart pain

Causes include:

- Abnormalities of the heart valves
- Excessive use of stimulants such as alcohol, cocaine and caffeine, among others
- Heart attach
- Heart muscle disease (cardiomyopathy)
- High blood pressure
- Hypertrophy
- Ischemia

EKG characteristic of Atrial Flutter include:

- A regular rhythm during which the AV node conducts impulses to the ventricles at a 2:1, 3:1, or 4:1 ratio. Occasionally, a greater ratio can be identified. The rhythm is variable to the AV blocks which may be consistent or variable.
- Fast heart rate: 250 – 350 bpm.

- Presence of flutter waves. Some are buried in the QRS complex.
- P-QRS ratio: mostly 2:1, sometimes 3:1 or 4:1.
- Variable PR intervals.
- QRS complex forms usually normal: 0.06 – 0.10 seconds. Some QRS complexes may appear wider if flutter wave is buried in QRS.

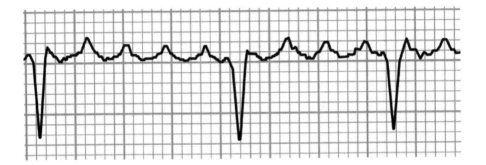

Management for Atrial Flutter includes:

- For rate control:
  - Administration of beta blockers, calcium channel blockers, and digoxin
  - Cardioversion
  - Arrhythmic medications for rhythm control
  - Rapid atrial pacing
- Radiofrequency ablation (RFA) for atypical flutter
- Catheter-based ablation for first-line patients with typical atrial flutter type 1

Atrial flutter is most common in elderly clients and clients with heart disease. It is also important to note that clients with atrial flutter carry the same stroke risk as clients with atrial fibrillation.

5. *Atrial Fibrillation (AF or A-fib)*

Atrial fibrillation is an abnormal heart rhythm which results in rapid and irregular breathing. It is less common than atrial flutter. It is caused by the extreme excitability of atrial tissue. Both unifocal and the multifocal atrial tachycardia can develop into an irregularly irregular rhythm referred to as atrial fibrillation. As mentioned earlier, although normally discharged by the sinus node, every cell in the heart is capable of initiating an impulse. In atrial fibrillation, atrial activity is chaotic and the AV node is bombarded with impulses at 300 bpm. This chaotic electrical activity results in an irregularly irregular pattern on EKG. In atrial fibrillation, the intervals on EKG are completely random because the ventricles are not paced by any one side.

Symptoms include:

- Chest pain
- Dizziness
- Exercise intolerance
- Fatigue
- Feeling of palpitations
- Shortness of breath

Causes include:

- Coronary artery disease
- Excessive alcohol intake
- Heart valve problems
- Hypertension
- Obesity
- Sleep apnea
- Thyroid disease

EKG characteristics of Atrial Fibrillation include:

- An irregular rhythm which is caused by the erratic and rapid discharge which emanates from multiple atrial foci.
- Absence of an organized atrial depolarization.
- Fast heart rate of up to 350 bpm.
- Absence of distinguishable P waves.
- No P-QRS ratio.
- No PR intervals.
- Normal QRS complex forms: 0.06 – 0.10 seconds.

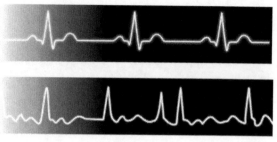

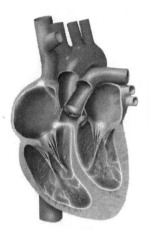

Atrial Fibrillation

Management for Atrial Fibrillation includes:

- Administration of beta blockers, calcium channel blockers, or digoxin for rate control
- Anticoagulation in clients who are in risk of developing a stroke from atrial fibrillation
- Cardioversion to treat fast or irregular heartbeat
- Radiofrequency ablation (RFA)
- Recommend lifestyle changes, such as cutting back on salt intake, a healthy diet, reducing stress, and limiting stimulants such as alcohol, caffeine, and smoking

6. *Review Question & Rationale:*

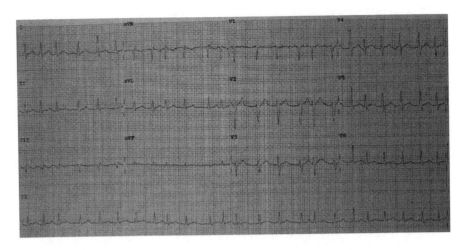

The nurse notes the above on the EKG monitor strip. The nurse should anticipate an order for which of the following medications?

     a. Acetaminophen (Tylenol)

     b. Aspirin (ASA)

     c. Ibuprofen (Motrin)

     d. Indomethacin (Indocin)

Answer B is correct. The EKG strip indicates atrial fibrillation with a heart rate of around 150 bpm. Clients who experience this irregular rhythm are at risk of developing blood clots. Because of this, anticoagulants such as aspiring are to be administered in order to prevent an ischemic stroke due to clot formation. Answer A, C, and D are all incorrect because the NSAIDS listed are not usually given to patients who are at risk of clot formation.

Section 6-C: Ventricular Arrhythmias

There are three main types of ventricular arrhythmias which include the following:

- Premature ventricular contractions (PVCs)
- Ventricular tachycardia (VT)
- Ventricular fibrillation (VT)

These arrhythmias range from benign to life-threatening and will be discussed in this subsection.

1. *Premature Ventricular Contractions (PVCs)*

Premature beats which are initiated from the ventricle are called premature ventricular contractions (PVCs). In terms of irregularity, PVCs follow the same principle as PACs. PVCs are caused by tissue in the ventricles that discharge electrical impulses erratically and irregularly.

- If every other heat beat is premature, this is called **ventricular bigeminy.**
- If every third heart beat is premature, this is called a **ventricular trigeminy.**

PVCs can be both unifocal and multifocal in nature. Unifocal and isolate PVCs, which will have the same appearance throughout any given lead, are usually benign. Multifocal PVCs are different in appearance from one another and are a common indication of an underlying heart disease.

Although PVCs are commonly benign, the presence of PVCs in an indication there there is some form of irritability in the ventricles and it is therefore important to identify whether the PVC is benign or serious (thereby potentially life-threatening) and also whether it has the potential to cause lifestyle-limiting symptoms.

When assessing PVCs, the following factors should be noted:

- Unifocal vs multifocal appearance
- Symptomatic vs asymptomatic
- Frequency of PVCs
- Presence vs absence of structural cardiac abnormalities

PVCs often do not cause any symptoms, although the following sensations are sometimes encountered:

- An increased awareness of one's heartbeat
- Fluttering
- Irregular heart beat
- Palpitations
- Pounding

- Shortness of breath
- Skipped/missed beats

Causes include, but are not limited to:

- Certain drugs, such as asthma medication and digoxin
- Chemical changes or imbalances in the body
- Excessive adrenalin
- Excessive intake of alcohol or drugs
- Excessive use of stimulants such as alcohol, caffeine or tobacco
- Underlying heart disease or scaring

On EKG, a PVC is usually followed by a full compensatory pause. This is because the sinus node timing is not interrupted, thereby firing off the next impulse on time.

EKG characteristics of PVCs include:

- An irregular rhythm whenever a PVC occurs.
- A rate which depends on the underlying rhythm.
- No P waves.
- P-QRS ratio: no P waves
- No PR intervals.
- Wide and bizarre QRS complex of greater than 0.1 seconds.

The diagram below shows a PVC marked by an arrow.

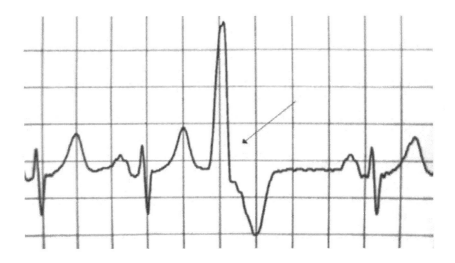

Management of PVCs:

- Lifestyle changes, e.g. reducing intake of caffeine and tobacco
- Administration of medications such as beta blockers and calcium channel blockers
- Radiofrequency ablation (RFA)

2. *Ventricular Tachycardia (VT)*

A run of three or more consecutive PVCs is called ventricular tachycardia. VT is representative of AV dissociation with atrial and ventricular impulses occurring entirely independent of one another. Because of this, the presence of AV dissociation is diagnosis of VT. The ventricular rate, which in VT is usually always faster than the atrial rate, is usually between 120 and 200 bpm.

VT can be uniform (monomorphic) or polymorphic. Uniform VT are similar in appearance with all beats. Polymorphic VT vary in appearance from beat to beat. A polymorphic VT indicates that there is more than one irritable area in the heart. Uniform VT is most commonly encountered in healed infarctions. Polymorphic VT is most commonly associated with acute coronary ischemia and/or infarction.

VT should be classified as sustained or non-sustained. If the VT is sustained, i.e. it lasts for longer than 30 seconds, it requires urgent and immediate treatment.

Brief VT is usually asymptomatic but if longer-lasting it can cause symptoms such as:

- Chest pain
- Dizziness
- Light-headedness
- Near-fainting or fainting
- Palpitations
- Shortness of breath
- Weak or no pulse

Common causes of VT include:

- Electrolyte imbalances
- Increased automaticity
- Prolonged QT interval
- Scarring, e.g. after an infarction or after heart surgery
- Underlying heart problems such as coronary artery disease, high blood pressure, heart valve disease or cardiomyopathy
- VT is most commonly a complication that arises from ischemic heart disease or left ventricular dysfunction

EKG characteristics of monomorphic VTs include:

- A regular rhythm.
- A fast heart rate: 100 – 250 bpm.
- No P waves.
- P-QRS ratio: no P waves
- No PR intervals.
- Wide and bizarre QRS complex of greater than 0.1 seconds. QRS complexes nevertheless have the same shape and amplitude, i.e. they are monomorphic.

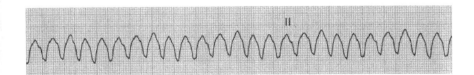

EKG characteristics of polymorphic VTs include:

- A regular or irregular rhythm.

- A fast heart rate: 100 – 250 bpm.
- No P waves.
- P-QRS ratio: no P waves
- No PR intervals.
- Wide and bizarre QRS complex of greater than 0.1 seconds. Variation in the shape and amplitude of QRS complexes.

Treatment for a client with stable VT is tailored to that specific client. If VT becomes an emergency situation, e.g. pulseless VT or unstable VT, immediate treatment is required.

Treatment includes:

- Immediate cardioversion if the client still has a pulse
- Electrical defibrillation if the client is pulseless
- Administration of anti-arrhythmic medications
- Surgery in some cases

3. *Torsades De Pointes*

This is a form of polymorphic VT that is especially unstable. Torsades de pointes, or twisting of the points, can quickly degenerate into ventricular fibrillation. Torsades are most commonly encountered in the presence of prolonged QT intervals. Its most common causes include electrolyte abnormalities, certain medications, and genetic variations. On EKG, the QRS reverses polarity and exhibits a spindle effect (twisting) around the baseline.

.

EKG characteristics of Torsades de pointes include:

- An irregular rhythm.
- A fast heart rate: 200 – 250 bpm.
- No P waves.
- P-QRS ratio: no P waves
- No PR intervals.
- Wide and bizarre QRS complex of greater than 0.1 seconds.

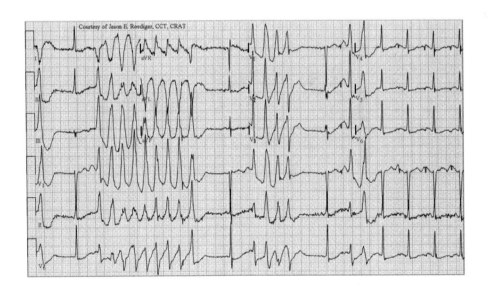

4. _Ventricular Fibrillation (VF)_

Unlike VT, there is no organized activity in the ventricles in clients with ventricular fibrillation. There is no identifiable pattern on EKG: no P wave, no QRS complex, no T wave. In VF, the heart generates no cardiac output and immediate electrical defibrillation and cardiopulmonary resuscitation are required. VF often occurs with cardiac arrest and is a common cause in clients with sudden cardiac death.

EKG characteristics of monomorphic VTs include:

- A chaotic rhythm.
- An indeterminate hear rate
- No P waves, no PR intervals, no QRS complexes

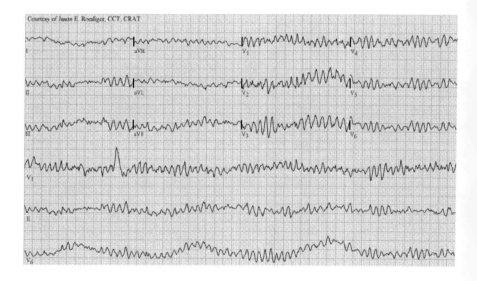

Untreated VF will lead to asystole. Asystole, or cardiac standstill, is the complete cessation of electrical activity of the heart and ultimately leads to cardiac death.

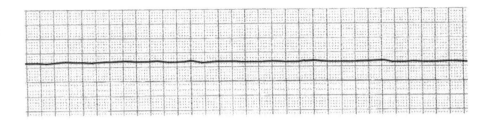

5. *Review Question & Rationale*

The nurse notes the following on the EKG strip. The nurse evaluates the client to be experiencing which of the following arrhythmias?

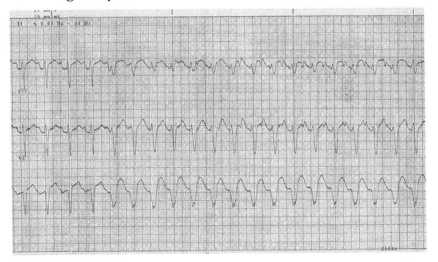

    a. A sinus rhythm
    b. Atrial fibrillation

c. Atrial flutter

d. Ventricular tachycardia

Answer D is correct. The EKG strip shows ventricular tachycardia. Answers A, B, and C are all incorrect because these are not noted on the EKG strip.

Section 7: Determining the Axis

The EKG records the vector of electrical conduction at any given moment. The axis is the general direction of the electrical conduction through the heart, i.e. it represents the average direction of the current flow. As covered in *Section 4,* each lead represents a different angle of orientation. All of these added together represent one average QRS vector, which we call the axis.

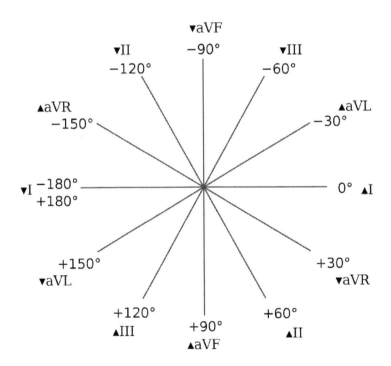

The QRS complex represents ventricular depolarization. Each lead represents a depolarization vector within the heart. As we can recall from *Section 4* and the diagram below, Lead I separates negative and positive angles from one another. Everything above Lead I is negative because the impulse here spread downwards. Everything below Lead I is positive because the impulses that are discharged from here travel upwards.

1. _The Four Quadrants_

Depending on their axis, each client will fall into one of four categories: normal, intermediate, left, or right. Whether the client's axis is left, right, normal, or indeterminate, is determined based on the four quadrants.

- **Normal Axis:** If the QRS vector lies within 0 and +90 degrees, the EKG has a normal axis (NML). The NML points points down and to the client's left.
- **Right Axis Deviation:** If the QRS vector lies within +90 and +180 degrees, the EKG has a right axis deviation (RAD). The right axis points down and to the client's right side.
- **Left Axis Deviation:** If the QRS vector lies within 0 and -90 degrees, the EKG has a left axis deviation (LAD). The left axis points down and to the patient's left.
- **Indeterminate Axis:** The indeterminate axis is an extreme axis deviation which falls between -180 and -90 degrees. Whenever the QRS lies in the indeterminate axis, it is important to check the client

for lead misplacement or possible ventricular tachycardia.

The four quadrants are created by the intersection of Lead I (which runs from the left arm to the right arm) and Lead aVF (which runs from the head to the feet), which intersect the heart's center.

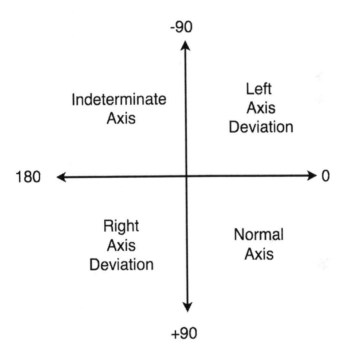

2. *Method for Determining the Axis*

The axis quadrant can be easily determined using Lead I and Lead aVF. It is important to remember that Lead I and Lead aVF are both positive on one side and negative on the other. Lead I is positive on the left hand and negative on the right arm. Lead aVF is positive at the feet and negative at the head.

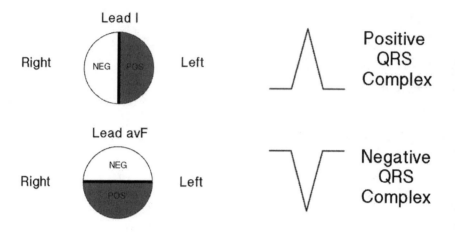

In order to determine the electrical axis of the heart, use the following pointers:

- **NMD:** If the axis falls into the lower left quadrant (to the client's left and near the feet), making Leads I and aVF both positive, the axis is normal. The QRS complex in both Lead I and Lead aVF will be positive.

- **Indeterminate:** On the contrary, if the QRS deflection is negative in both leads (pointing to the client's head and to the right), the axis will be indeterminate.

- **RAD:** If the axis falls in the lower right quadrant, the axis is in the right axis deviation (positive in Lead aVF and negative in Lead I). The QRS complex in Lead I will be negative, but it will be positive in Lead aVF.

- **LAD:** If the axis however falls within upper left quadrant, then the axis is in the left axis deviation (negative Lead aVF and positive Lead I). The QRS complex in Lead I will be positive, but it will be negative in Lead aVF.

Any QRS vector which is orientated between -90 and +90 degrees (in the LAD and NML quadrants), will produce a WRS complex which is predominantly positive in Lead I. Any QRS vector which lies between 0 and 180 degrees will produce a QRS complex which is predominantly positive in Lead aVF.

Lead aVF

		Positive	Negative
	Positive	Normal Axis	LAD
Lead I			
	Negative	RAD	Indeterminate Axis

In summary, if the QLS is positive in both leads, the axis is normal. If it is positive in Lead I and negative in Lead aVF, the axis is LAD. If it is negative in Lead I and positive in Lead aVF, the axis is RAD.

It will usually be sufficient to note whether the axis is normal (NML) or not. However, it is possible to be more precise and to actually determine the exact degree of the axis. You can determine the approximate axis using the following degrees: 0, 30, 60, 90, 120, 150, and 180 which are marked in the diagram below.

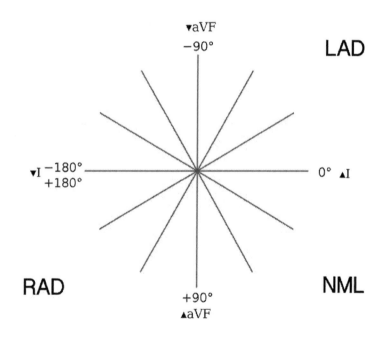

3. *Defining the Electrical Axis of the Heart Precisely:*

In order to determine the axis in degrees, follow the steps

below:

1. Determine the quadrant the axis falls into (NML, LAD, RAD, or indeterminate).
2. Determine which lead is most isoelectric, that is, the lead with equal force in the positive and negative direction. The esoteric lead is usually the lead with the smallest QRS complex.
3. From the isoelectric lead, move 90% degrees towards the quadrant which you identified in Step 1.

So for example, if Lead I is positive and Lead aVF, your axis is in the NML (Step 1). Then determine your isoelectric lead. If your QRS complex in Lead III is smallest, of equal force in the positive and negative direction, or biphasic, this will be your isoelectric lead (Step 2). Now move 90% degrees towards the quadrant identified in Step 1 (NML) (Step 3). Your axis is at an angle of +30 degrees!

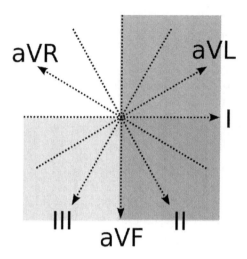

4. *Abnormal Heart Axis*

In the normal heart, the QRS axis lies somewhere between 0 and 90 degrees. Significantly, an abnormal electrical axis of the heart can provide indications as to the presence of heart injury or a complication pertaining to the conduction system, such as heart block, infarction, ischemia, or hypotrophy.

Obesity for example, which increases the abdominal tissue, can cause left axis deviation. On the other hand, people with a tall and thin frame, can develop right axis deviation, which is caused by the heart stretching vertically. Some pulmonary diseases also cause right axis deviation by hyperinflation of the lungs which also stretches the heart vertically.

Common causes of LAD:

- Inferior myocardial infarction
- Left anterior fascicular block (hemiblock)
- Left bundle branch block
- Left ventricular hypertrophy
- Obesity
- Paced rhythm
- Ventricular ectopy
- Wolff-Parkinson White syndrome

Common causes of RAD:

- A tall and thin body frame
- Acute lung disease, such as PE
- Chronic lung disease, such as COPD
- Hyperkalaemia
- Lateral wall myocardial infarction
- Left posterior fascicular block
- Right bundle branch block
- Right ventricular hypertrophy
- Sodium-channel blocker toxicity
- Ventricular ectopy
- WPW syndrome

Section 8: Heart Block

Heart block occurs when there is a delay in the normal flow of electrical impulses which results in the heart beating too slowly. To recap what was covered in *Section 1,* conductions are normally initiated in the sinus node and then spread through to atria to the AV node, to the bundle of His, before splitting into the right and left bundle branches through the ventricles. Defined by their respective anatomic location, there are different types of conduction blocks:

- Sinus node block
- AV block
- Bundle branch block

Common causes of heart block include the following:

- Administration of certain types of medicines, including beta-blockers, calcium channel blockers, and digoxin
- Complication of Lyme disease
- Endocarditis (Infection of the heart valves)
- Hemochromatosis
- Myocardial infarctions
- Sarcoidosis
- Scarring (fibrosis) of the heart's electrical conduction system. This is often caused by aging and is the most common cause of heart block

The picture below displays in circles the main sites of the three conduction blocks. In this section, we will cover the following heart blocks: sinus pause/arrest, AV blocks, right and left bundle branch block, and right and left hemiblock.

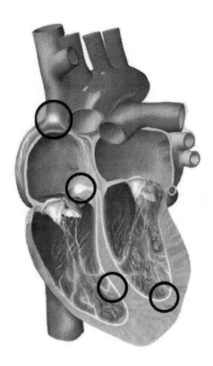

Section 8-A: Sinus Node Block

1. *Sinus Arrest/Sinus Pause:*

Sinus arrest or sinus pause is a condition in which the sinus node ceases to discharge electrical impulses. Sinus arrest is diagnosed by the absence of the P wave. Because the heart contains several pacemakers, the pause usually only last a few seconds.

EKG characteristics include:

- An irregular rhythm that occurs whenever there is a sinus pause, due to the SA node failing to discharge impulses for a prolonged period, then resumes impulse initiation.
- A heart rate which varies between normal to slow depending on the duration of the sinus arrest.
- Normal P waves which are upright and uniform (apart from during pause).
- Normal PR intervals: 0.12 – 0.20 seconds.
- Normal QRS complex: 0.06 – 0.10 seconds.

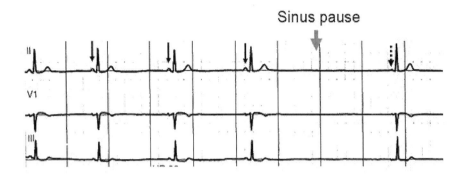

Sinus pause

2. *Sinus Block*

A sinus block occurs when the electrical impulse is blocked on its way to the atria. Most sinus blocks do not require treatment.

EKG characteristics include:

- An irregular rhythm that occurs whenever there is a sinus block. The block results in a dropped beat after which the rhythm continues regularly until the next sinus block occurs.
- A heart rate which varies between normal to slow depending on how frequent sinus blocks occur.
- Normal P waves which are upright and uniform (apart from during the block).
- Normal PR intervals: 0.12 – 0.20 seconds.
- Normal QRS complex: 0.06 – 0.10 seconds.

Section 8-B: AV Block

An atrioventricular (AV) block occurs when there is a delay in the electrical impulse of the heart as it spreads from the atria to the ventricles.

Causes of AV block include:

- Aging
- Ischemic heart disease
- Heart rate-slowing medications, including beta blockers, calcium channel blockers, digoxin, and antiarrhythmic medications
- Electrolyte abnormalities, particularly potassium
- Cardiac surgery (AV block being a possible complication)

There are four types of AV heart blocks:

- First-degree AV block
- Second-degree AV block (Mobitz type I)
- Second-degree AV block (Mobitz type II)
- Third-degree AV block (complete heart block)

1. ***First-Degree AV Block***

A first-degree AV block is not a blockage as such, but instead a delay in the conduction of the impulse form the sinus node to the AV node which is represented by a prolonged PR interval on EKG. Depolarization spreads as usual from the sinus node through the atria but when reaching the AV node, instead of passing through immediately, the impulse is held up for bit before passing through the AV node. As a result of this, the PR interval is prolonged. The first-degree AV block is the mildest form of heart block and generally does not produce any symptoms. It is an occurrence that often comes with aging, as well as a result of hear rate-slowing medications or ischemia.

EKG characteristics include:

- A regular rhythm.
- A heart rate which depends on the underlying rhythm.
- Normal P waves which are upright and uniform.
- Prolonged PR interval greater than 0.2 seconds
- Normal QRS complex: 0.06 – 0.10 seconds

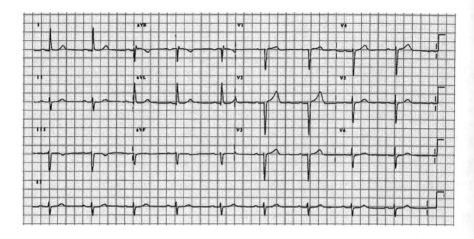

The EKG above shows a left anterior fascicular block and a first-degree heart block, which is characterized by a prolonger PR interval (greater than 0.2 seconds). The rhythm is sinus and the QRS is a left ward axis (below -30 degrees).

First-degree AV block does not require any treatment by itself. The presence of first-degree AV block does however raise the risk of other heart rhythm problems, such as atrial fibrillation. Should the client experience any symptoms or is taking rate-slowing medications, it is important to monitor and document the PR interval on EKG.

2. *Second-Degree AV Block Type I (Mobitz Type I)*

In second-degree AV block, not every impulse manages to

pass through the AV node. There are two different types of second-degree AV blocks: Mobitz type I (also called the Wenckebach block) and Mobitz type II. It is crucial to make a distinction between the two because Mobitz type II is more severe than Mobitz type I. A Mobitz type I block is usually caused by a conduction bloc in the AV node. It is usually benign and very rarely degenerates to third-degree heart block. Mobitz type II heart block is usually caused by a conduction block below the AV node, near the bundle of His. It is a more serious heart block which is capable of suddenly degenerating to a third-degree heart block. Treatment is usually not required for a Mobitz type I block. In contrast, a Mobitz type II block usually requires the insertion of a pacemaker.

SECOND-DEGREE AV BLOCK TYPE I (MOBITZ TYPE I OR WENCKEBACH).

The Mobitz type I AV block is defined by a PR interval which becomes progressively longer from cycle to cycle before a dropped QRS complex. The beat occurs when the AV node is no able to conduct an impulse from above. The interval which follows the beat is significantly shorter, as can be seen on the EKG strip below.

Because this AV block occurs in the AV node, the QRS complex (which represents the electrical conducting through the ventricles), will usually appear normal. When identifying a Mobitz type I second-degree AV block, it is important to pinpoint the beat which is followed by a shortened PR interval.

Mobitz type I EKG characteristics include:

- Atrial rhythm is regular, ventricular rhythm is irregular.
- A heart rate which depends on the underlying rhythm.
- Normal P waves which are upright and uniform with overall more P waves than QRS complexes.
- Progressively lengthening PR interval until one P wave is entirely blocked and id therefore not followed by a QRS complex. The cycle is eventually repeated after a pause, during which the AV node recovers).
- Normal QRS complex: 0.06 – 0.10 seconds.

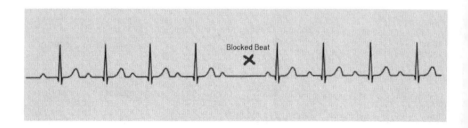

Mobitz type I does not produce any specific symptoms and rarely requires treatment. It is common in young and healthy people and often occurs during sleep. It is nevertheless important to monitor this type of heart block if it is persistent because Mobitz type I AV block can sometimes degenerate to more severe forms of heart block.

3. *Second-Degree AV Block Type II (Mobitz Type II)*

The Mobitz type II AV block is usually caused by a block below the AV node in the bundle of His. This is a less common, but more serious type of heart block. Like Mobitz type I, only some atrial impulses are transmitted through to the ventricles. The PR interval is however not progressively lengthened. On EKG, you will instead spot two or more normal PR intervals with a P wave which is not followed by a QRS complex (a dropped beat). The dropped beat is unpredictable and often inconsistent. This results in a ratio of P waves to QRS complexes which is rarely constant (varying between 2:1 to 3:2 to 4:1, and so on). Because this block occurs lower down in the electrical conduction system, the QRS complex will usually be wide. All these factors make this type of heart block more unstable and more serious.

Mobitz type II EKG characteristics include:

- Atrial rhythm is regular, ventricular rhythm is either regular or irregular.
- Atrial heart rate of 60 – 100 bpm and a ventricular heart rate which is slower than the atrial rate
- Normal P waves which are upright and uniform with overall more P waves than QRS complexes. The ratio

(P waves to QRS complexes) is often 2:1, 3:1, 4:1, or variable.

- Constant PR intervals which are either normal or prolonged
- QRS complexes are often wide, that is, longer than 0.10 seconds

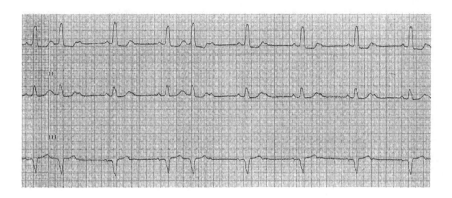

The EKG above shows a Mobitz type II AV block with a left bundle branch block in conducted beats. In essence, the Mobitz type II heart block is defined by punctual P waves which are constant in cycle length and which are sometimes followed by a QRS complex, sometimes not. It is important to not confuse Mobitz type II blocks with a blocked PAC (a premature P wave that is not followed by a QRS complex – please refer back to *Section 6* for more information).

4. *__High Grade AV Block / 2:1 AV Block__*

This is also a form of second-degree AV block, which is characterized by the absence of every second QRS complex, that is, two or more P waves that are not followed by QRS complexes. This essentially means that for every two atrial impulses, there is only ventricular impulse. Every type of 2:1 AV block is referred to as a 'high-grade heart block'. If the 2:1 block is hemodynamically unstable or causes symptoms, a temporary or permanent pacemaker should be inserted. The EKG strip below shows a sinus rhythm with a 3:2 and 2:1 Type 2 AV block.

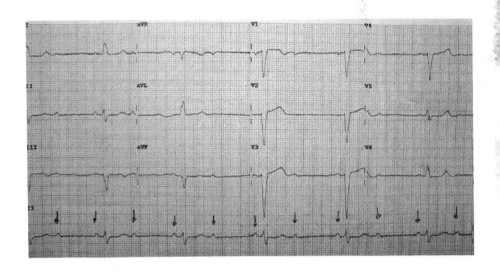

5. *Third-Degree AV Block / Complete Heart Block*

A third-degree AV block or complete heart block occurs when no atrial depolarization can pass through the AV node. The complete electrical block between the atria and the ventricles is called 'AV dissociation'.

AV dissociation refers to the situation in which the atria and the ventricles are driven by separate pacemakers (the atria continues to contract at its intrinsic rate of 60 to 100 bpm whereas the ventricles contract at their own intrinsic rate which is 40 to 45 bpm). The block is either located in the AV node or slightly lower. As a result of this, the ventricles generate a junctional escape rhythm at a rate of typically 30 to 45 bpm.

EKG characteristics of third-degree AV block include:

- The rhythm is usually regular with the atria and the ventricles acting independently.
- Atrial heart rate of 60 – 100 bpm and ventricular contraction rate of 40 – 60 bpm.
- Normal P waves which are upright and uniform but which are at times superimposed on QRS complexes or T waves.
- Great variations in the PR intervals.
- QRS complexes will be normal if the ventricles have activated their junctional escape focus, otherwise wide.

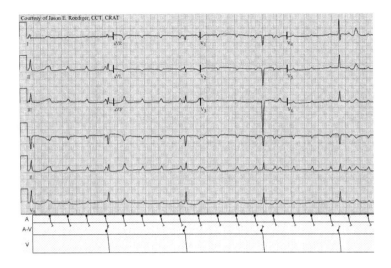

The EKG strip above shows sinus tachycardia with a
complete AV block and resulting junctional escape. On V6
(the 6th line), you can see that the P waves are present but
that no QRS complexes follow.

**It is important to note that the diagnosis of a complete
heart block requires the presence of AV dissociation.** This
can be identified by a ventricular rate which is slower than
the atrial or sinus rate. When diagnosing a third-degree AV
block, you should also identify the location of the escape
focus. Identify the QRS complex – the slower and the wider
it is, the lower the block in the conduction system. The lower
down the block, the more unstable it is. It is important to
interpret the entire EKG because patients with third-degree
AV block require urgent and immediate care - the insertion
of a permanent pacemaker is generally required. Complete
heart block can also develop prenatally and can cause

symptoms such as fainting and lightheadedness.

Lastly, it is important to mention that the different degrees of AV block can exist in the same patient and that one degree of AV block can degenerate into another. A patient may for example have a first-degree AV block, as well as a Mobitz type I block. A patient with a Mobitz II block can at a later stage also develop a complete heart block.

Section 8-C: Bundle Branch Block

Delays in ventricular conduction occurs when ventricular depolarization takes longer than 0.1 seconds. On EKG, the QRS complex will appear wider than two to three small boxes. Hemiblocks (incomplete right bundle branch block, left anterior fascicular block, or left posterior fascicular block) often results in a QRS duration of 0.1 to 0.12 seconds, whereas a complete bundle branch block is represented by a QRS duration which is greater than 0.12 seconds.

In order to understand the effect of bundle branch blocks, it is important to review ventricular depolarization. In a normal heart beat, the electrical impulse spreads through the AV node into the left and right bundle and down the ventricles. This causes the ventricles to contract almost simultaneously. If there is a delay in one bundle branch, this will slow down conduction in that area. The unblocked bundle branch will therefore contract sooner and depolarize the surrounding heart muscle, which leads to passive depolarization of the other ventricle with the blocked bundle branch. On EKG, this is represented by a wide QRS complex. In general, the more extensive the bundle branch block, the wider the QRS will appear on EKG. The length of the QRS reflects the length of the time it takes for passive depolarization of one ventricle to travel across the septum.

The diagnosis of bundle branch block is made by examining the width as well as the configuration of the QRS complexes.

EKG characteristics of bundle branch block include:

- A regular rhythm.
- A heart rate that depends on the underlying rhythm.
- Normal P waves which are upright and uniform.
- Normal PR intervals: 0.12 – 0.2 seconds.
- QRS complexes which are wide (greater than 0.12 seconds) and which are sometimes have a notched appearance (rabbit ears).

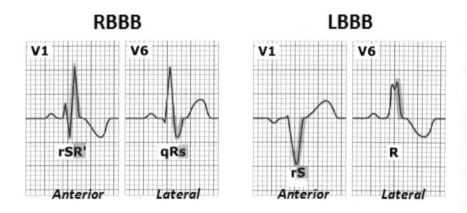

In order to diagnose a bundle branch block, the first step is to identify a QRS complex which is longer than 0.12 seconds in duration. The second step is to examine Lead V1 and Lead V6 in order to differentiate between RBBB and LBBB.

1. *Right Bundle Branch Block (RBBB)*

Right bundle branch block (RBBB) occurs when the conduction through the right bundle is obstructed. This results in a delay in right ventricular depolarization. The right bundle only starts to depolarize once the left ventricle is almost fully depolarized.

The following are EKG characteristics which are specific to RBBB:

- Right axis deviation is often seen clients with RBBB (see previous section).
- R prime (R, R′) pattern which is most visible in **Lead V1 and Lead V2** (sometimes also in Lead V3) – the R wave represents left ventricular activation and the R′ represents right ventricular activation (see diagram below).
- **In Lead V6,** the tall R wave represents left ventricular activation. Right ventricular activation is represented by the small S (see diagram above).

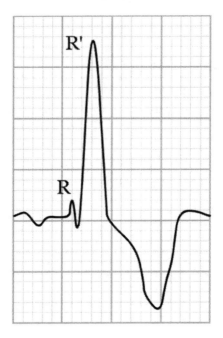

The EKG strip below shows a sinus rhythm with a 3:1 and 2:1 Type II AV block and a right bundle branch block, which can be identified in Lead V1 and Lead V6.

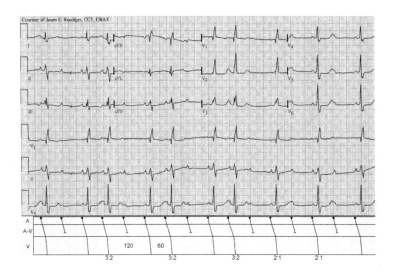

Common causes of RBBB include:

- Aging – RBBB is particularly associated with fibro-calcific conduction disease
- Atrial septal defect
- Pulmonary arterial hypertension
- Pulmonary embolus
- Pulmonary stenosis
- Right ventricular hypertrophy

When caring for a patient with RBBB, it is important to monitor for for first-degree AV block and for left hemiblock. This is because in the presence of other heart blocks, the potential for RBBB to degenerate to complete heart block is more significant.

2. *Left Bundle Branch Block (LBBB)*

Although left bundle branch block (LBBB) also causes a very wide QRS complex on EKG, it is entirely different in appearance when compared to RBBB. LBBB causes the right ventricle to depolarize first. The left bundle only starts to depolarize once the right ventricle is almost fully depolarized.

The following are EKG characteristics which are specific to LBBB:

- Left axis deviation is often seen clients with LBBB (see previous section).
- In **Lead V1**, the QS complex represents the slow of ventricular depolarization from the right bundle to the left bundle, the Q representing right ventricular depolarization and the S representing left ventricular depolarization.
- In **Lead V6** there will be a tall R wave instead and no q wave (usually a R, R′ pattern). The R represents right ventricular activation and the R′ represents left ventricular activation.
- Inverted T waves are sometimes also seen on EKG in the presence of LBBB.

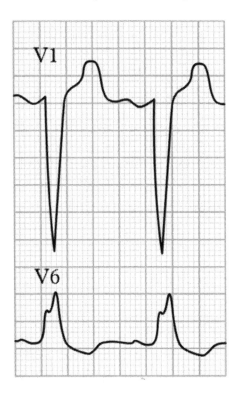

Unlike RBBB, LBBB is more often associated with structural heart disease, in particular, coronary artery disease and valvular heart disease. The presence of LBBB also renders the diagnosis of ischemia on EKG more difficult. In the presence of LBBB, it is always important to examine the patient's EKG for other conduction delays. This is because the presence of other heart blocks, such as incomplete right bundle branch block (IRBBB) or first-degree AV block, can significantly increase the patient's risk for third-degree heart block. It is also important to assess the patient's drug history, particularly for any antiarrhythmic medications or rate-slowing medications, and review any medications that could potentiate heart block disease.

3. *Right and Left Bundle Hemiblock (IRBBB, LAFB, and LPFB)*

If the duration of the QRS complex is greater than 0.1 seconds but lower than 0.12 seconds, then this is a potential indication of a hemiblock. There are three different types that we will discuss in this section:

- Incomplete right bundle branch block (IRBBB) – Right Bundle Hemiblock
- Left anterior fascicular block (LAFB) – Left Bundle Hemiblock
- Left posterior fascicular block (LPFB) – Left Bundle Hemiblock

There are three types of hemiblocks because as covered in *Section 2* of this guide, the right bundle branch comprises of only one fascicle, whereas the left bundle branch consists of two: an anterior fascicle and a posterior fascicle. In order to help you visualize the location of the block, we have included then image below which you will remember from *Section 2*. You will also remember that number 5 is the left posterior fascicle, number 6 is the left anterior fascicle, and number 10 is the right bundle branch.

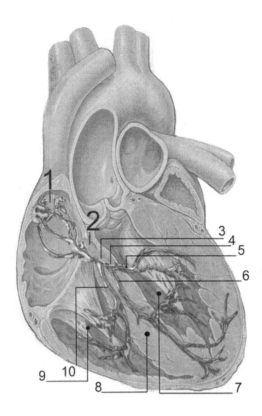

When dealing with a left bundle hemiblock, it is crucial to distinguish between a LAFB and a LPFB. As we mentioned in *Section 4,* it is crucial to remember the different lead groups. Unless you have already memorized these groups, I would recommend you revisit this section as this is key in the diagnosis of left bundle hemiblocks.

Incomplete RBBB (IRBBB)

On EKG, the IRBBB will have a similar appearance to the complete right bundle branch block, but with a shorter QRS duration (of less than 0.12 seconds). Right axis deviation is often also present.

Left Anterior Fascicular Block (LAFB)

This type of hemiblock, which is located near the anterolateral portion of the left ventricle, is much more common than a LPFB.

In the presence of LAFB, there is a left axis deviation of -30 to -45 degrees, or sometimes more negative. There are two main clues on EKG which are key in the diagnosis of LAFB:

- rS pattern in the inferior leads
- qR pattern in the lateral leads

Left Posterior Fascicular Block (LPFB)

This hemiblock is located near the right side of the left ventricle and therefore results, if blocked, in a right axis deviation of +120 degrees, or more positive. The EKG findings for LPFB (which are the opposite to that seen on EKG for LAFB) include the following:

- qR pattern in the inferior leads
- rS pattern in the lateral leads

In *Section 5* of this book I have said that there are five main areas that you need to master in order to effectively interpret EKG: rate, rhythm, axis, block and infarction. We have now covered the first four. In the next and last substantive section, we will now discuss ischemia and infarctions.

4. *Review Question:*

The nurse has been assigned to a client who has been admitted to the emergency unit with shortness of breath, anxiety, and tachycardia. The EKG reveals that the client is suffering from atrial fibrillation with a ventricular heart rate of 130 bpm. The physician prescribes quinidine sulfate. Whilst administering the medication, which of the following should the nurse monitor in EKG?

    a. Elevated ST segment
    b. Inverted T wave
    c. Peaked P wave
    d. Prolonged QT interval

Answer D is correct. The nurse should monitor the client's QT intervals, because quinidine can cause widened Q-T intervals as well as heart block. Other EKG signs of toxicity include widened QRS complexes and notched P waves. The most common side effects of the medication include vomiting, diarrhea and nausea, but the client may also experience signs of confusion, headache, visual disturbance, and vertigo. Answer A, B, and C are all incorrect because these EKG changes are not associated with quinidine.

Section 9: Myocardial Ischemia and Infarction

Ischemia: Ischemia is the restriction in blood supply to the tissues which results in decreased blood flow and tissue hypoxemia. This decrease in blood flow causes delays in the heart's depolarization and repolarization pattern. If ischemia spreads across the entire thickness of the ventricular wall, there is an imminent danger of myocardial infarction.

Infarction: Infarction is the complete obstruction of one of the coronary arteries, which restricts a tissue's blood supply, thereby causing a lack of depolarization tissue death.

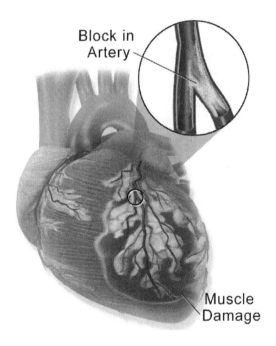

Block in Artery

Muscle Damage

1. *Using EKG to Diagnose an Evolving Ischemia and Infarction*

There are several stages of an ischemia and infarction which can be traced on EKG. In this part, we will cover the three main changes of an evolving infarction which are visible on EKG:

1. **T wave which peaks and then inverts:** An **inverted T wave** is associated with the initial stages of Ischemia.

In diagram below shows a normal T wave that is tall and upright in shape. With the onset of an infarction, the T wave becomes even taller – a phenomenon which is called 'peaking.'

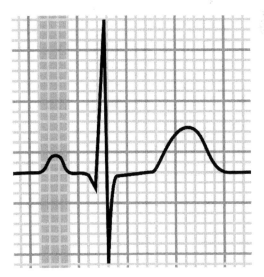

A couple of hours later, the T wave inverts in the same patient. The diagram below shows an inverted T wave. These changes in T waves are representative of an ischemia – a lack of adequate blood flow to the heart muscle.

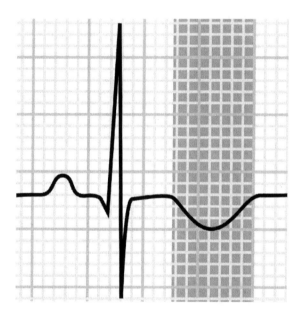

It is important to note that the inverted T wave is only representative of an ischemia and is not per se diagnostic of infarction. On top of this, there are other conditions that can cause an inverted T wave, such as bundle branch blocks.

2. __ST segment depression, followed by a ST segment elevation__

- **ST segment depression** will be visible on EKG as the ischemia extends into the deeper layers of the myocardium – **ST depression is an indicator that an infarction may be imminent.**
- **ST segment elevation** reflects myocardial injury. Elevation of the ST segment above the baseline is called the **injury pattern** and is representative of early-stage infarction. It is suggestive of cellular damage beyond ischemia.

As we recall from *Section 3* of this book, the ST segment is the horizontal baseline immediately before the the T wave. The diagram below shows a normal ST segment on EKG which is highlighted by the vertical strip. In general, a depression or elevation with a deflection of 2 small boxes or more should be considered to be clinically significant.

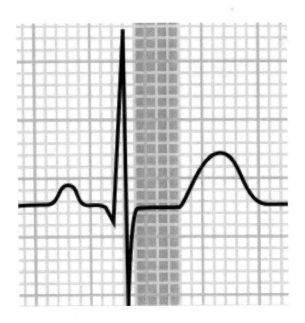

3. Q wave/the first downward deflection after the P wave is indicative of an infarction.

The appearance of new Q waves is an indication of infarction. By this time, the ST segment has usually returned to the baseline.

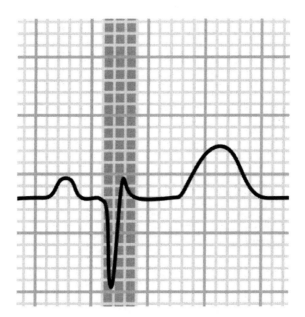

The new Q waves tend to persist forever in clients who have suffered from myocardial infarction. Scar tissue after a myocardial infarction does not depolarize. Because of this, once an area of the myocardium has died, it becomes electronically silent. Electrical vectors will then point away from this area. Any electrodes overlying the dead tissue will record a deep negative deflection. On EKG therefore, infarctions are presented by negative forces, that is, Q waves and inverted T waves (as highlighted in the diagram above).

Leads that are located near the infarction site will experience an increase in electrical activity that is directed toward them. These leads will record positive and tall R waves. These opposing changes, which are called **reciprocal changes**, are recorded by distant leads. These distant leads will record a ST segment depression.

On the EKG strip below, the highlighted sections marked with a X show ST segment elevation in Leads I, aVL, and V1 to V5 with reciprocal changes (highlighted and marked with O) in the inferior leads. These EKG findings are indicative of anterior wall myocardial infarction.

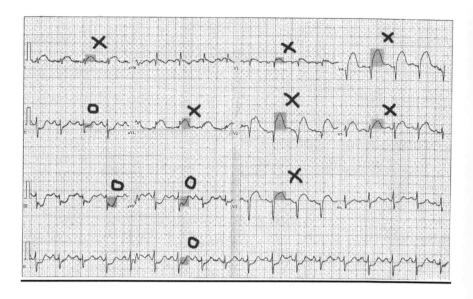

2. *Normal Vs. Pathologic Q Wave*

In normal hearts, a small Q wave can be seen in the left lateral leads and sometimes also in the inferior leads. In comparison, pathologic Q waves which are indicative of infarction are wider and deeper in form. Because of this, they are often referred to as **significant Q waves.** In general, the EKG criteria for pathologic Q waves include the following:

- A Q wave which is longer than 0.04 seconds in duration (i.e. longer than one small box on EKG paper).
- The depth of the Q wave is at least one third the height of the R wave in the same QRS complex.

The diagram below shows a pathologic Q wave:

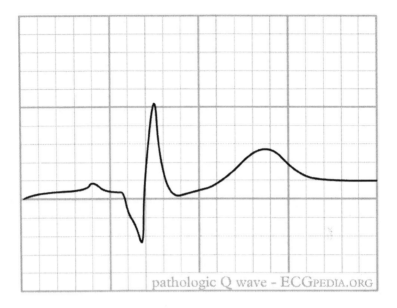

pathologic Q wave - ECGPEDIA.ORG

3. *Coronary Blood Supply to the Conduction System*

The following are the main coronary arteries:

The right coronary artery (RCA) supplies blood to the **inferior wall** (EKG Leads: II, III, aVF), more specifically to the:

- Sinus node (supplied by the conal branch of the RCA)
- AV node
- Right ventricle
- Inferior portion of the left ventricle

The left anterior descending artery (LAD) supplies blood to the <u>anterior wall</u> (EKG Leads: V1, V2, V3, V4), more specifically to the:

- Right and left bundle branch (supplied by the perforating branches of the LAD)
- Interventricular septum
- Anterior portion of the left ventricle

The left circumflex artery supplies blood to the <u>lateral wall</u> (EKG Leads: I, aVL, V5, V6), more specifically to the:

- Lateral wall of the left ventricle
- Sinus node (less common)
- AV node (less common)

Depending on which artery is dominant, either the RCA or the left circumflex artery supply blood to the **posterior wall.**

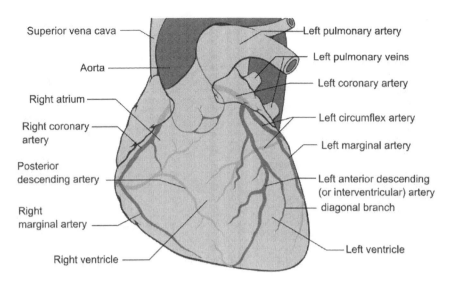

Superior vena cava — Left pulmonary artery

Aorta — Left pulmonary veins

Left coronary artery

Right atrium —

Right coronary artery — Left circumflex artery

Left marginal artery

Posterior descending artery —

Right marginal artery — Left anterior descending (or interventricular) artery

diagonal branch

Right ventricle — Left ventricle

4. *Locating the Infarct*

When diagnosing ischemia or infarction, it is very important to follow a pattern: begin by examining the inferior leads, the lateral leads, and then the anterior leads. Examining them in their groups is important in terms of helping you narrow down the focus of the affected area. Also recall which main coronary artery supplies this section.

Leads	Group
Leads V1, V2, V3, V4	Anterior chest leads
Leads I, aVL, V5, V6	Left lateral leads
Leads II, III, aVF	Inferior leads
Lead aVR	-

It is important to note that if, for example, there is a Q wave in Lead II, but not in Lead III and Lead aVF, this should be interpreted as a 'non-specific finding.' It cannot be diagnostic of an old inferior wall myocardial infarction because in order for a diagnose an ischemia or infarction, there have to be changes in all contiguous leads.

When diagnosing ischemia or infarction, reciprocity is also something that should be kept in mind. Injury itself will be represented by ST elevation. The reciprocal change therefore will take the form of ST depression. In order to help confirm the diagnosis, it is again helpful to examine the leads as individual groups and to note the following:

- Reciprocal changes in the inferior leads is indicative of anterior wall injury and/or later wall injury.
- Reciprocal changes in the lateral leads is indicative of inferior wall injury.
- Reciprocal change sin the anterior leads is indicative of posterior wall injury.

Infarctions are grouped into several categories depending on the site of the infarct and include: anterior infarctions, inferior infarctions, lateral infarctions, and posterior infarctions.

ANTERIOR WALL ISCHEMIA & INFARCTION

Blood to the anterior myocardium is supplied by the left anterior descending artery. An ischemia affecting this area can be diagnosed by examining the T waves and the ST segments in the precordial chest leads (**Leads V1 to V4**). The following EKG characteristics are indicative of an ischemia affecting the anterior wall:

- **Reciprocal changes** in the inferior leads (Leads II, III, and aVF).
- Early stage ischemia is reflected by a **T wave inversion** in Leads V1 to V4.
- A progressing ischemia is reflected by a **ST segment depression** in Leads V1 to V4.
- Ongoing injury is reflected by **ST segment elevation** in Leads V1 to V4.
- Transmural infarction is reflected by **Q waves** in Leads V1 to V4.

The diagram below shows a myocardial infarction (labelled 2) of the anterior wall. This was caused by a blockage (labelled 1) of a branch of the left coronary artery (LCA).

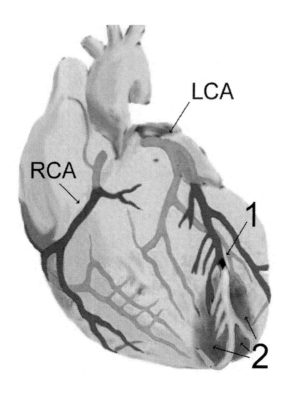

INFERIOR WALL ISCHEMIA & INFARCTION

Blood to the inferior myocardium is supplied by the RCA. An infarction in the inferior wall of the heart is commonly caused by an occlusion of the RCA or its descending branch. An ischemia affecting this area can be diagnosed by examining the T waves and the ST segments in the inferior leads leads (**Leads II, III, and aVF**). The following EKG characteristics are indicative of an ischemia affecting the inferior wall:

- **Reciprocal changes** in the left lateral leads (Leads I, aVL, V5, and V6).
- Early stage ischemia is reflected by a **T wave inversion** in Leads II, III, and avF.
- A progressing ischemia is reflected by a **ST segment depression** in Leads II, III, and avF.
- Ongoing injury is reflected by **ST segment elevation** in these leads.
- Transmural infarction is reflected by **Q waves** in the same leads.

Because the RCA also supplied the AV node, a complete heart block (third-degree heart block) is sometimes also associated with acute inferior wall infarction. A myocardial infarction in the inferior wall will often also result in left axis deviation with the electrical vectors pointing away from the infarct.

LATERAL WALL ISCHEMIA & INFARCTION

Blood to the lateral wall is supplied by the left circumflex artery. An ischemia affecting this area can be diagnosed by examining the T waves and the ST segments in the left lateral leads (**Leads I, aVL, V5, and V6**). The following EKG characteristics are indicative of an ischemia affecting the lateral wall:

- **Reciprocal changes** in the inferior leads (Leads II, III, and aVF).
- Early stage ischemia is reflected by a **T wave inversion** in Leads I, aVL, V5, and V6.
- A progressing ischemia is reflected by a **ST segment depression** in Leads I, aVL, V5, and V6.
- Ongoing injury is reflected by **ST segment elevation** in these leads.
- Transmural infarction is reflected by **Q waves** in the same leads.

A myocardial infarction in the lateral wall will often also result in right axis deviation because, as we discussed earlier, electrodes point away from the area of injury (which has become electronically 'silent').

POSTERIOR WALL ISCHEMIA & INFARCTION

An infarction in the posterior wall is rarely seen alone. Posterior wall infarction is most commonly observed in the presence of inferior or lateral wall infarction. Blood to the posterior wall is supplied by either the RCA or the left circumflex area (depending on which of the two supplies the majority of the posterior wall). Diagnosing an ischemia in this area is significantly more difficult because the placement of the leads in the classic 12-lead EKG does not provide a good view onto the posterior wall of the heart. As a result of this, we have to rely on reciprocal changes in the diagnosis of posterior wall ischemia and infarction.

Depolarization of the posterior wall is the exact opposite of depolarization of the anterior wall. Because of this, diagnosing an ischemia affecting the posterior wall is made by looking at the reciprocal changes in the anterior chest leads. As we discussed earlier, **anterior wall** infarction can be diagnosed by identifying a ST segment elevation and Q waves in the anterior chest leads (**Leads V1, V2, V3, and V4**). An ischemia in the posterior wall will produce a 'mirror image'. The following EKG characteristics are indicative of an ischemia affecting the posterior wall of the heart:

- Posterior wall ischemia is reflected by **tall R waves and ST segment depression** in the anterior leads (Leads V1 to V4).
- A progressing ischemia is reflected by the development of **larger S waves and smaller R waves** in Leads V1 to V4.

5. *EKG Limitations & Sgarbossa's Criteria*

As covered above, a typical diagnosis of an evolving myocardial infarction includes ST segment changes as well as the appearance of a new Q wave. An underlying cardiac condition can however distort EKG findings, which makes diagnosis by way of EKG interpretation unreliable. Right bundle branch blocks (RBBBs) do not usually alter EKG findings of ischemia or infarction. Left bundle branch blocks (LBBBs) on the other hand, affects both phases of ventricular depolarization and is thereby represented by Q waves, St segment, the loss of normal R wave progression, as well as T wave changes. All these EKG findings can also be present in ischemia and infarction. Nevertheless, there are specific criteria that can be used to diagnose an ischemia or infarction in the presence of LBBB.

Sgarbossa's criteria are a set of EKG findings can be used to diagnose a suspected infarction the presence of a LBBBs or ventricular paced rhythms. They include the following:

- **ST elevation >1 mm in leads with a positive QRS complex** – QRS concordant with ST segment (score 5)
- **ST depression >1 mm in Leads V1, V2, and/or V3** (score 3)
- **ST elevation >5 mm in leads with a negative QRS complex** – QRS discordant with ST segment (score 2)

It is important to note that although these criteria are sensitive, they are not specific for myocardial infarction. A total score of > 3 is said to to have a specificity of 90% for diagnosing infarction.

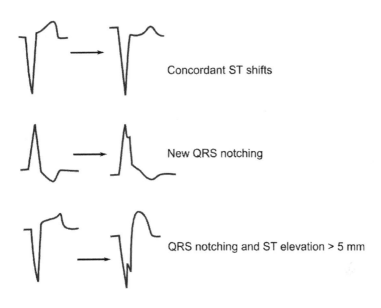

Concordant ST shifts

New QRS notching

QRS notching and ST elevation > 5 mm

6. *Review Question & Rationale*

The nurse has been assigned to the client with substernal chest pain radiating to the left jaw who has been admitted to the emergency unit. Which of the following EKG findings suggests to the nurse that the client may experience acute myocardial infarction?

    a. Changes in ST segment

    b. Minimal QRS wave

    c. Peaked P wave

    d. Prominent U wave

Answer A is correct. Changes in ST segment is a EKG

finding that is indicative of acute myocardial infarction. Answer B, C, and D are all incorrect because minimal QRS waves, peaked P waves, and prominent U waves are not associated with acute infarction of the heart.

Section 10: Final Notes

I would like to take this opportunity to thank you for purchasing this book. I hope you now have a solid foundation, and that this guide has helped you equip yourself with the knowledge for achieving success with the EKG interpretation.

My final piece of advice - no matter how diligent you are in your studies, your best learning will come from proactively testing your knowledge. I recommend revisiting any sections and questions that you have found difficult to constantly refresh and build on your knowledge as you progress.

I sincerely wish you the best of luck in your nursing career.

Best wishes,

Eva Regan

33000636R00074

Made in the USA
Middletown, DE
25 June 2016